THE DIABETES BOOK:

A GUIDE TO MANAGING TYPE 2 DIABETES

BY CAROL HARRELL

COPYWRIGHT TEMPLATE

TABLE OF CONTENTS

CHAPTER 1:

About type 2 diabetes

Who is at greater risk of developing type 2 diabetes?

Symptoms of type 2 diabetes

CHAPTER 2:

Causes of type 2 diabetes

CHAPTER 3:

Risk factors and complications

CHAPTER 4:

Prevention and management

How can I keep my type 2 diabetes under control?

CHAPTER 5:

Treatment, medications and diet for type 2 diabetes

CHAPTER 6:

Receiving diagnosis for type 2 diabetes

Children with type 2 diabetes

Statistics on type 2 diabetes

The impact of diabetes

CHAPTER 1

ABOUT TYPE 2 DIABETES

The most common form of diabetes, type 2, is a condition in which your blood glucose, also known as blood sugar, is too high. Blood glucose, which comes primarily from food, is your primary energy source. The pancreas makes insulin, a hormone that helps glucose get into your cells and be used for energy. In type 2 diabetes, your body doesn't make adequate insulin or doesn't use insulin well. After that, your blood contains too much glucose, and not enough reaches your cells.

Chronically, high blood glucose levels caused by uncontrolled type 2 diabetes can result in a number of symptoms and serious complications. However, the good news is that you can take steps to reduce or prevent type 2 diabetes from developing.

Who is at greater risk of developing type 2 diabetes?

Type 2 diabetes can occur at whatever stage in life, even in youth. However, people in their middle and later years are more likely to develop type 2 diabetes. If you are over 45, have a family history of diabetes, are overweight, or are obese, you are more likely to get type 2 diabetes. African Americans, Hispanic/Latino, American Indians, Asian Americans, and Pacific Islanders are more likely to develop diabetes.

Your risk of developing type 2 diabetes is increased by physical inactivity and certain health issues like high blood pressure. If you have prediabetes or had gestational diabetes while pregnant, you also have a greater risk of developing type 2 diabetes.

Symptoms of type 2 diabetes

In type 2 diabetes, your body can't really utilize insulin to bring glucose into your cells. This makes your body to depend on sources of elective energy in your tissues, muscles and organs. This is a chain response that can cause many side effects.

The signs and symptoms of type 2 diabetes frequently grow gradually. As a matter of fact, you can be living with type 2 diabetes for quite a long time and not know it. At the point when signs and side effects are available, they might include:

-Expanded thirst

-Continuous pee

-Expanded hunger

-Accidental weight reduction

-Exhaustion

-Obscured vision

-Slow-mending injuries

-Consistent yearning

-Absence of energy

-Incessant diseases

-Numbness or shivering in the hands or feet

-Areas of obscured skin, for the most part in the armpits and neck

As the sickness advances, the side effects become more serious and can cause a few possibly perilous inconveniences. In the event that your blood glucose levels have been high from now onward, indefinitely quite a while, the signs can include:

-eye issues (diabetic retinopathy)

-sensations of deadness in your limits or neuropathy

-kidney sickness (nephropathy)

-gum sickness

-coronary failure or stroke

When to see a specialist

See your Primary Care Physician (PCP) on the off chance that you notice any signs of type 2 diabetes.

Type 2 diabetes- the most common type of diabetes - is caused by a number of factors, including lifestyle factors and characteristics.

- **Overweight, corpulence, and actual dormancy:**

You are bound to develop type 2 diabetes in the event that you are not active physically and are overweight or have heftiness. Additional weight once in a while causes insulin opposition and is normal in individuals with type 2 diabetes. The area of muscle to fat proportion moreover has an effect. Insulin resistance, type 2 diabetes, and heart and vein disease are all linked to additional stomach fat.

- **Insulin opposition:**

Type 2 diabetes typically starts with insulin obstruction, a condition in which muscle, liver, and fat cells don't utilize insulin well. As a result, your body requires more insulin to facilitate glucose entry into cells. From the get go, the pancreas makes more insulin to stay aware of the additional increase. Over time, blood glucose levels rise when the pancreas is unable to produce enough insulin.

- **Genes and family ancestry:**

As in type 1 diabetes, certain qualities might make you bound to develop type 2 diabetes. The illness generally affects families, but it occurs more frequently in these racial/ethnic groups:

o African Americans

o The Frozen North Locals

o Native Americans

o Asian Americans

o Hispanics/Latinos

o Local Hawaiians

o Pacific Islanders

Genes likewise can Increase the risk of type 2 diabetes by increasing an individual's propensity to become overweight or have stoutness.

CAROL HARRELL

CHAPTER 3

RISK FACTORS AND COMPLICATIONS

Risk factors

Factors that might build your risk of type 2 diabetes include:

- **Weight:** Being overweight or hefty is a fundamental risk.

- **Fat circulation:** Putting away fat basically in your midsection — as opposed to your hips and thighs — shows a more serious risk. Your risk of type 2 diabetes rises on the off chance that you're a man with a midsection perimeter over 40 inches (101.6 centimeters) or a lady with an estimation over 35 inches (88.9 centimeters).

-**Inactivity:** The more inactive you are, the more your risk. Active exercise aids in weight management, converts glucose into energy, and makes your cells more susceptible to insulin.

-**Family ancestry:** The risk of type 2 diabetes increases assuming your parent or kin has type 2 diabetes.

                    CAROL HARRELL

-Race and nationality: Despite the fact that it's not clear why individuals of specific races and identities — including Dark, Hispanic, Local American and Asian individuals, and Pacific Islanders — are bound to develop type 2 diabetes than white individuals are.

-Blood lipid levels: A high risk is related with low levels of high-density lipoprotein (HDL) cholesterol (the good cholesterol) and greater levels of fatty substances.

-Age: The risk of type 2 diabetes increases as you progress in years, particularly after age 45.

-Prediabetes: Prediabetes is a condition where your glucose level is higher than typical, yet not sufficiently high to be delegated diabetes. If left untreated, prediabetes frequently advances to type 2 diabetes.

-Pregnancy-related chances: Your risk of having type 2 diabetes increases in the event that you had gestational diabetes when you were pregnant or on the other hand assuming that you brought forth a child who weighed more than 4 kilograms.

-Polycystic ovary disorder: Having polycystic ovary condition — a typical condition portrayed by sporadic feminine periods, overabundance hair development and weight — builds the risk of diabetes.

-Areas of obscured skin, typically in the armpits and neck: This condition frequently shows insulin obstruction.

-Eating a ton of highly processed foods: Highly processed food varieties can have a great deal of stored away sugar and refined carbs.

On the off chance that your life requires a more "in and out" kind of eating style, talk with your PCP or a dietician about nourishment swaps.

Complications

Type 2 diabetes impacts numerous critical organs, including your heart, nerves, veins, eyes and kidneys.

Likewise, factors that increase the risk of diabetes are risk factors for other serious ongoing illnesses. Managing diabetes and controlling your glucose level can bring down your risk for these inconveniences or existing together circumstances (comorbidities).

Possible complications of diabetes and successive conditions include:

-Heart and vein infection: Diabetes is related with a high risk of coronary illness, stroke, hypertension and limiting of veins (atherosclerosis).

-Nerve damage (neuropathy) in appendages: High glucose over the long run can harm or obliterate nerves, bringing about shivering, deadness, consuming, torment or possible loss of feeling that generally starts at the tips of the fingers or toes and gradually moves upward.

-Other nerve damages: Damage to nerves of the heart can add to unpredictable heart rhythms. Nerve damage in the stomach related framework can create some issues with nausea, diarrhea, constipation or vomiting. For men, nerve damage might cause erectile brokenness(dysfunction).

-Kidney infection: Diabetes might prompt constant kidney sickness or irreversible end-stage kidney illness, which might require dialysis or kidney transplant.

-Eye damage: Diabetes increases the risk of serious eye sicknesses, like waterfalls and glaucoma, and may harm the veins of the retina, possibly prompting visual deficiency.

-Skin conditions: Diabetes might leave you more helpless to skin issues, including bacterial and parasitic contaminations.

-Slow healing: Cuts and rankles can become serious contaminations, which might slowly heal if left untreated. Extreme harm could require toe, foot or leg removal.

-Deficit in hearing: Diabetes patients are more likely to experience hearing problems.

-Sleep apnea: Obstructive sleep apnea is normal in individuals living with type 2 diabetes. Diabetes might be the super contributing component to the two circumstances. It's not confirmed if treating sleep apnea further improves glucose control.

-Dementia: Type 2 diabetes appears to increase the risk of Alzheimer's sickness and different issues that cause dementia. Poor control of glucose levels is connected to a high decrease in memory and other reasoning abilities.

Others include:

-Stroke

-Respiratory failure: Ladies with diabetes are bound to have a respiratory failure, at a more youthful age, than ladies without diabetes.

Men with diabetes are 3.5 times as liable to develop erectile dysfunction.

-Hypoglycemia: Hypoglycemia can happen when your glucose is low. The side effects can incorporate flimsiness, wooziness, and trouble talking. You can typically cure this by having a "convenient solution" food or refreshment, similar to natural product juice, a soda, or hard treats.

-Hyperglycemia: Hyperglycemia can happen when glucose is high. It is ordinarily described by continuous pee and increased thirst. Observing your blood glucose cautiously, and remaining active, can assist with forestalling hyperglycemia.

-Inconveniences during and after pregnancy:

Assuming you have diabetes while you're pregnant, you'll have to carefully monitor your condition. Diabetes that is ineffectively controlled may:

-complicate pregnancy, labor, and delivery

-hurt your child's developing organs

-make your child put on overabundant weight

-It can likewise increase your child's risk of developing diabetes during their lifetime.

CHAPTER 4

PREVENTION AND MANAGEMENT

Even if you have biological relatives who are living with diabetes, making healthy lifestyle choices can help prevent type 2 diabetes. Changes in your lifestyle may slow or stop the progression to diabetes if you have been diagnosed with prediabetes.

Included in a healthy lifestyle are:

-Eating nutritious foods: Choose foods that are higher in fiber and lower in calories and fat. Concentrate on whole grains, vegetables, and fruits.

-Getting in shape: Aim for 150 minutes or more per week of moderate-to-vigorous aerobic exercise, such as swimming, biking, walking, or cycling.

-Weight loss: The transition from prediabetes to type 2 diabetes can be slowed down by maintaining a modest weight loss. Losing 7% to 10% of your body weight can lower your risk of developing diabetes if you have prediabetes.

-Avoiding prolonged periods of inactivity: Long periods of sitting can raise your risk of type 2 diabetes. Try to get up and move around for at least a few minutes every thirty minutes.

How can I keep my type 2 diabetes under control?

                    CAROL HARRELL

Type 2 diabetes can be effectively managed by controlling blood glucose, blood pressure, and cholesterol levels, as well as by quitting smoking if you smoke. Diabetes management also includes making lifestyle changes like planning healthy meals, limiting calories if you're overweight, and getting active. Likewise, taking any prescribed medications. Create a diabetes treatment plan that works for you by working with your medical team.

CHAPTER 5

TREATMENT, MEDICATIONS AND DIET FOR TYPE 2 DIABETES

TREATMENT FOR TYPE 2 DIABETES

Type 2 diabetes can be managed, and in some cases, reversed, with treatment. Your doctor will tell you how often you should check your blood glucose levels as part of the majority of treatment plans. The objective is to maintain a certain range.

To assist in the treatment of type 2 diabetes, your doctor may recommend the following additional lifestyle modifications:

- Eating fruits, vegetables, and whole grains, which are high in fiber and healthy carbohydrates, on a regular basis can help maintain steady blood glucose levels.

- learning to pay attention to your body's signals and when to stop eating.

-Control your weight and maintain heart health by avoiding refined carbohydrates, sweets, and animal fats as much as possible.

Get at least 30 minutes of exercise every day to maintain heart health. Exercise can also help regulate blood glucose levels.

                                    CAROL HARRELL

MEDICATIONS FOR TYPE 2 DIABETES

In some instances, lifestyle adjustments are sufficient to control type 2 diabetes. If not, there are a number of medications that may be of assistance. Among these medications are:

-**Metformin:** Your body's response to insulin may be enhanced and blood glucose levels may be decreased as a result. For the majority of people with type 2 diabetes, it is the first line of treatment.

-**Sulfonylureas:** These are pills that your body takes orally to make more insulin.

-**Meglitinides:** These medications stimulate your pancreas to release more insulin and have a short half-life.

-**Thiazolidinediones:** Your body is more sensitive to insulin because of these.

-**Inhibitors of dipeptidyl peptidase 4 (DPP-4):** These are milder drugs that assist with decreasing blood glucose levels.

- **Glucagon-like peptide-1 agonists:** These slow down digestion and improve glucose levels in the blood.

-**Inhibitors of the sodium-glucose cotransporter-2 (SGLT2):** These assist your kidneys in eliminating sugar from your body via urine.

Side effects can occur with any of the above-mentioned medications. Finding the best diabetes medication or medication combination may take some time for you and your doctor.

                          CAROL HARRELL

You may require medication to address your cholesterol or blood pressure levels as well if they are not ideal.

You might need insulin therapy if your body doesn't make enough insulin. It's possible that all you need is a long-acting injection that you can take at night, or it's possible that you need to take insulin multiple times a day.

DIET FOR TYPE 2 DIABETES

The diet is an important tool for maintaining safe blood glucose levels and optimal heart health.

The eating regimen suggested for individuals with type 2 diabetes is a similar eating regimen basically everybody ought to follow. It all boils down to a few crucial steps:

- Select a variety of foods that are low in empty calories and high in nutrients.

- Work on controlling your portion sizes and deciding when to stop eating.

-Read food labels carefully to find out how much sugar or carbohydrates are in each serving.

Foods and Drinks To Limit

If you have type 2 diabetes or are trying to avoid it and control your weight, you should limit certain foods and drinks if at all possible. These are some:

- food sources high in saturated or trans fats (like red meat and full-fat dairy items)

- handled meats (like wieners and salami)

- margarine and shortening - refined baked goods (such as white bread and cake)

- high-sugar, highly processed snacks (such as packaged cookies and some cereals)

- sweet drinks (such as regular soda and some fruit juices)

 While no one food, enjoyed occasionally, ought to throw you off your healthy path, it's best to talk with your doctor concerning restrictions in diet based on the levels of your blood sugar. After consuming these foods, some individuals may require more careful glucose monitoring than others.

Foods to Choose

Having type 2 diabetes does not mean that carbs are out of the question. Carbohydrates that are healthy can give you energy and fiber. Among the options are:

-Whole fruits

-non-starchy vegetables like broccoli, carrots, and cauliflower

-legumes like beans

-whole grains like oats and quinoa

-sweet potatoes

All contain fat. Instead, selecting the appropriate fats is the key.Omega-3-rich foods include the following:

-tuna

-sardines

-salmon

-mackerel

-halibut

-cod

-flax seeds

Healthy monounsaturated and polyunsaturated fats can be found in the following foods:

-oils, like olive oil

-nuts, like almonds, pecans, and walnuts

-avocados

Discuss your individual dietary objectives with your physician. They might suggest that you talk to a dietitian who knows a lot about the best diets for diabetes. Together, you can devise a diet plan that complements your lifestyle and tastes great.

CHAPTER 6

RECEIVING DIAGNOSIS FOR TYPE 2 DIABETES

How do medical professionals diagnose this condition?

Blood tests can help your doctor figure out if you have type 2 diabetes.

If you think you might be experiencing signs of diabetes, you should see a doctor right away, regardless of whether you have prediabetes or not. Blood tests can provide your doctor with a lot of information. Examples of diagnostic procedures include:

-A1C hemoglobin test: The average blood glucose levels over the previous two to three months are measured by this test. This test does not require you to fast, and your doctor can make a diagnosis based on the results. A glycosylated hemoglobin test is another name for it.

-Fasting plasma glucose test: The amount of glucose in your plasma is measured by this test. Before taking it, you may need to fast for eight hours.

                                    CAROL HARRELL

- Test for oral glucose tolerance: Your blood is taken three times during this test: before, one hour, and two hours after you consume a glucose dose. The experimental outcomes show how well your body manages glucose when taken.

If you have diabetes, your doctor will give you the following advice on how to control it:

- how to monitor blood glucose levels on your own

- suggestions for diet and exercise

- information about any medications you need

You might need to see an endocrinologist who specializes in diabetes treatment. In the beginning, you probably need to go to the doctor more often to make sure your treatment plan is working.

CHILDREN WITH TYPE 2 DIABETES

The prevalence of type 2 diabetes among children is rising. The American Diabetes Association (ADA) estimates that 193,000 Americans under the age of 20 suffer from either type 1 or type 2 diabetes.

According to a 2016 study, the annual incidence of type 2 diabetes among youth has increased to approximately 5,000 new cases. Another 2017 study found a significant rise, particularly among racial and ethnic minority groups.

Before recommending a specific treatment, your child's doctor will need to determine whether they have type 1 or type 2 diabetes.

You can lower your child's risk by encouraging them to eat well and exercise every day, just as lifestyle choices can help adults manage or even reverse their type 2 diabetes diagnosis.

STATISTICS ON TYPE 2 DIABETES

The following information about diabetes in the United States is provided by the Centers for Disease Control and Prevention (CDC):

-Diabetes affects more than 30 million people. That amounts to roughly 10% of the population.

-One person in four is unaware that they have diabetes.

- 84.1 million adults have diabetes, but 90% of them are unaware of it.

-Black, Native American, and Hispanic adults who are not Hispanic are approximately twice as likely to have diabetes as white adults who are not Hispanic.

The following data are reported by the ADA:

-Diabetes resulted in lower productivity and direct medical costs totaling $327 billion in the United States in 2017.

-Compared to people who don't have diabetes, the average cost of medical care for diabetics is about 2.3 times higher.

-Diabetes is the seventh most common cause of death in the United States, either as the cause of death itself or as a factor in the death of a loved one.

The following information is provided by the WHO's Trusted Source:

- Adults worldwide had a prevalence of 8.5% of diabetes in 2014.

- Only 4.7% of adults worldwide had diabetes in 1980.

-In 2016, diabetes directly accounted for approximately 1.6 million deaths worldwide.

-Adults with diabetes have a nearly tripled chance of having a heart attack or stroke.

-Additionally, diabetes is a major contributor to kidney failure.

THE IMPACT OF DIABETES

                    CAROL HARRELL

The diagnosis of type 2 diabetes can be terrifying and overwhelming, and you probably have questions about why it developed, what it means for your long-term health, and how it will affect your day-to-day life.

You can get answers to your questions and learn more about what to expect from your doctor or nurse. They can likewise guide you to assets for clinical, as well as mental, support. These may include classes for groups; meetings with a nurse educator, social worker, or registered dietitian; and additional educational resources like magazines, websites, and books.

The majority of people experience emotional highs and lows for the first few months after being diagnosed. If you have just been given the news that you have diabetes, you and your family should make the most of this time to learn as much as you can so that taking care of your diabetes—such as testing your blood sugar, going to appointments, and taking your medications—will become part of your daily routine.

Complications with one's health, some of which can be serious, can result from type 2 diabetes. Be that as it may, there are things you can do to diminish your risk of fostering these issues.

The majority of people with diabetes continue to engage in a variety of activities and consume a variety of foods. Diabetes does not mean that "special occasion" foods like birthday cake are out of the question, and the majority of diabetics patients can and should enjoy almost any kind of exercise.